The Old Man From the Hill 2

(More Lessons in Qigong & Tai Chi)

By

Steve Zimcosky

Drawings and Cover Design by Jeromy Ko

Pictures of Dit Da Jow herbs and jar provided by East Meets West Intl. (eastmeetswest.com)

Pictures of Smock, Pennsylvania provided by the Smock Historical Society

(The journey continues from the first book, where a young boy has a chance encounter with an old Chinese man, who teaches him the ancient Chinese exercises of Qigong and Tai Chi. The lessons that he learned helped him with his health and other aspects of his life. Now in the following summer it is time to learn more.)

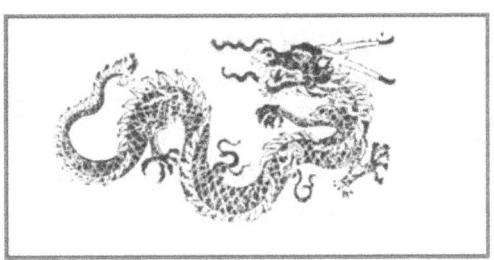

It was Friday May 27th, 1966 the day before the Memorial Day weekend. I was sitting in class at St. Stanislaus elementary school staring out the window. I was wondering if my mom and dad had decided to allow me to go stay with my grandparents for the upcoming summer. I was very excited to go and learn more from John. I had practiced everything that he taught me from the previous summer. I should have been more attentive to the math lessons because Sister Mary Joseph was calling on me to answer a question and I did not hear. Needless to say she got very upset with me.

When I got home somehow my mom knew I had gotten into trouble in school. She asked me why I was not paying attention in class. I explained how I was thinking of going back to Smock for the summer and that she and dad had not given me an answer yet. She told me to have patience. Patience was the one thing I was beginning to lose. There were only two more weeks of school left and I was very eager to learn more of what John had to teach.

On Sunday my parents took us to Bedford Reservation in the Metroparks for a Memorial Day picnic. It was the day before the holiday but my dad insisted the park would not be as crowded. He was wrong.

Mom and dad had found a nice secluded spot away from the crowds so we could have our family picnic. We all played wiffle ball, badminton, and other games while mom and dad got the grill and food set up. It was always fun playing with my siblings and then eating afterwards. Hot dogs, hamburgers and of course mom's potato salad was the menu for the picnic. It was

3

not what we were used to eating since we changed our diets according to what John had taught me. But it was a holiday and we thought, just this once it would be ok.

Everyone was tired when we got home as it was a long day of fun in the sun. Playing with my brothers and sisters the whole day made me forget about wanting to go back to Smock. I said good night to my mom and dad and it was then that they told me that I would be allowed to go back to smock. I was so excited that I could hardly sleep that night.

The next couple of weeks in school seemed like two months. I couldn't wait to go back and see John and learn more. My health and my self-esteem had become so much better. My grades had even improved to the point where the previous grading period I received straight A's and won tickets to a Cleveland Indians baseball game.

School ended on June 10th and I needed to wait until my dad could get his vacation to go to Smock. That meant waiting another week to go and it was driving me crazy.

Saturday, June 18th we were on our way to Smock. It was about a three hour trip on the Ohio and Pennsylvania turnpikes to get there. Once I saw the sign for state route 51 in PA. I knew we were just about there. I couldn't wait to see John and tell him how I practiced almost every day and how my life was so much better.

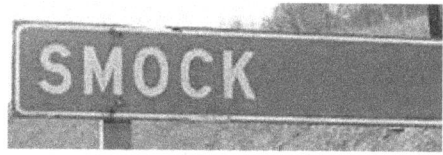

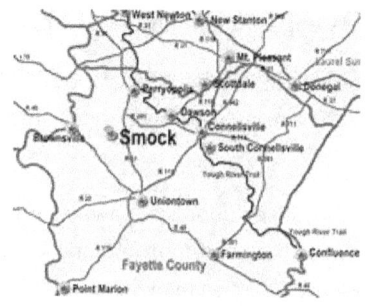

When we arrived at my grandparent's house I just wanted to take off up the hill to see John but that idea was cut short as my mom and dad wanted me to spend some time with my grandparents. It didn't matter though because they told me that John was away for the weekend visiting some friends in Pittsburgh. He would not return until Sunday night.

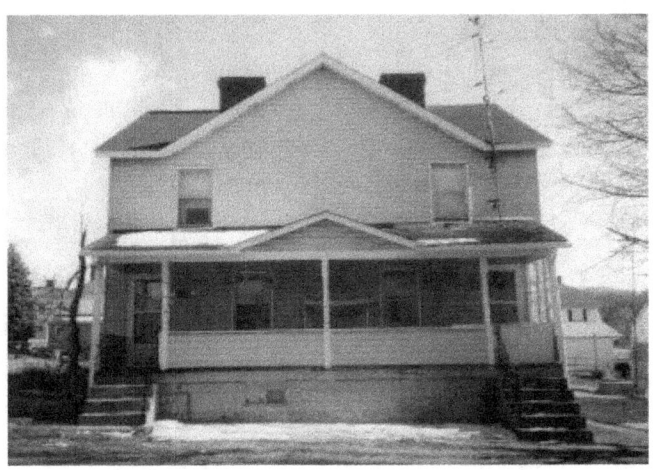

The weekend was nice and warm and sunny. I was able to play in their backyard with my brothers and sisters and cousins who had come by to visit us. It was a lot of fun but in the back of my mind I kept thinking of John.

My parents would be leaving on Monday to go home as my dad had some work to do around the house which was his reason for taking the vacation. I was glad I was staying because that meant I wouldn't have to help. I knew my brothers and sisters would be upset, they would be working and I would be having the fun.

Monday morning came real quick and my mom and dad finally got to meet John. They thanked him for teaching me and helping me to become healthier. They were glad that I had this opportunity to learn these exercises and how to take better care of myself. I hugged and kissed my mom and dad and just said goodbye to my brothers and sisters. We really didn't hug. We were like most kids in our neighborhood it just seemed to babyish to us.

As they pulled away I felt a sense of sadness and excitement at the same time. I was sad to see my family leave but I knew I would be learning more exercises from John. John turned to go up the hill to his little house and waved goodbye to my grandparents. I wasn't sure what to do since he didn't really say anything. Did I follow him or wait for him to ask me to go with him. A second later he turned to me and made a motion with his head that I should follow him.

We talked about how things had gone for each of us through the winter months, over tea. He was glad that I was so willing to come back and learn from him. He said that a lot of young people don't like the exercises because they seem so slow and boring. But I knew they were very beneficial; I was proof that they worked for good health.

He asked me to show him the exercises that I learned the previous summer and was happy to see that I was doing them very well. A daily practice, he said, is what keeps us healthy and full of energy. Before I knew it I had to go back to my grandparent's house for dinner. The time had gone by so quickly but I was really happy to there with John.

The next day I was up early, did my exercises and went downstairs to have breakfast with my grandparents. The sun was already coming up and it looked like it was going to be a beautiful day. As soon as I finished eating I asked my grandmother if she needed any help with the dishes and she said no. She knew how excited I was to get up the hill and start learning from John again. I was out the door in a flash and running up the hill.

As usual John was already up and doing his exercises in the open field. I never stopped being amazed at how gracefully he seemed to move for his age. It was like he was moving in slow motion. He also knew I was there watching him, as usual. I knew to wait until he was done before I said anything or went towards his house. It was the respectful thing to do.

He finished and motioned for me to come over to the house. John began to explain to me what I was going to learn this summer. I would be learning something called Fragrant Qigong, Chinese eye exercises, some new meditations and how to get Qi from nature. I reminded him about teaching me the short Tai Chi form I saw him do and he said that would come at the end of the summer.

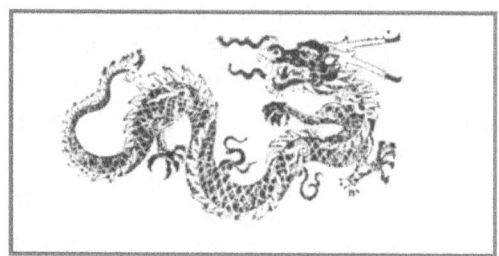

So we began. Fragrant Qigong, he explained, was a two thousand year old form of Qigong started by a Buddhist monk. It is called that because the more you practice this form of qigong the more you will notice a fragrant smell. He said that these exercises were the beginning level ones and would help the person practicing to be healthy, more energetic and even help people become smarter. The exercises he told me could be done while the person was in a car, on the phone, walking or even watching TV. It must be done while you are relaxed and with a smile. John had even taught this group of exercises to my grandparents.

The first movement is called the opening exercise. Start by placing your hands at chest level, facing each other without touching, and then separate them out and back five times. The hands should not touch.

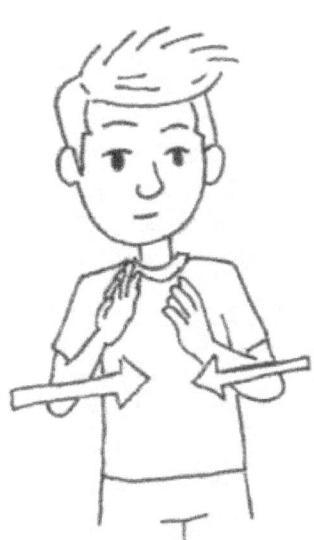 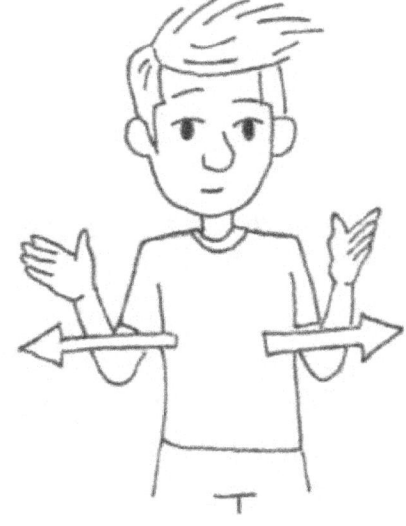

The next movement is called the tail. Your palms touch and then sweep down and up in a "U" shape. This helps to get your energy moving.

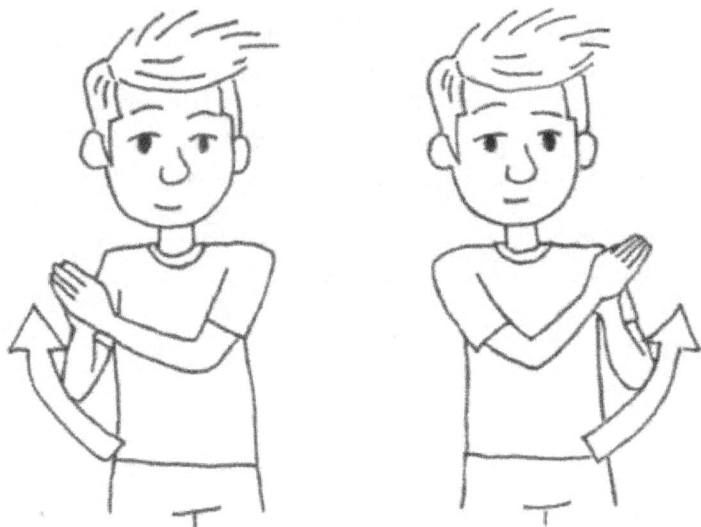

The next movement is called bird. Again the palms touch then you bring your elbows up so the hands come close to the chest and then back down. This helps to center your mind.

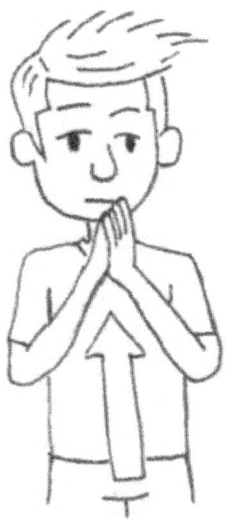
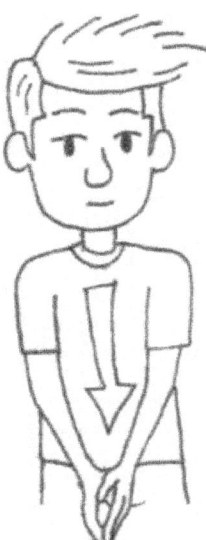

The next movement is called eight. Your hands are separated at chest level and facing each other. The hands sweep down and out to the sides of the body and then back to the starting position. Your palms should face the floor as the elbows go back. This calms your yang energy down.

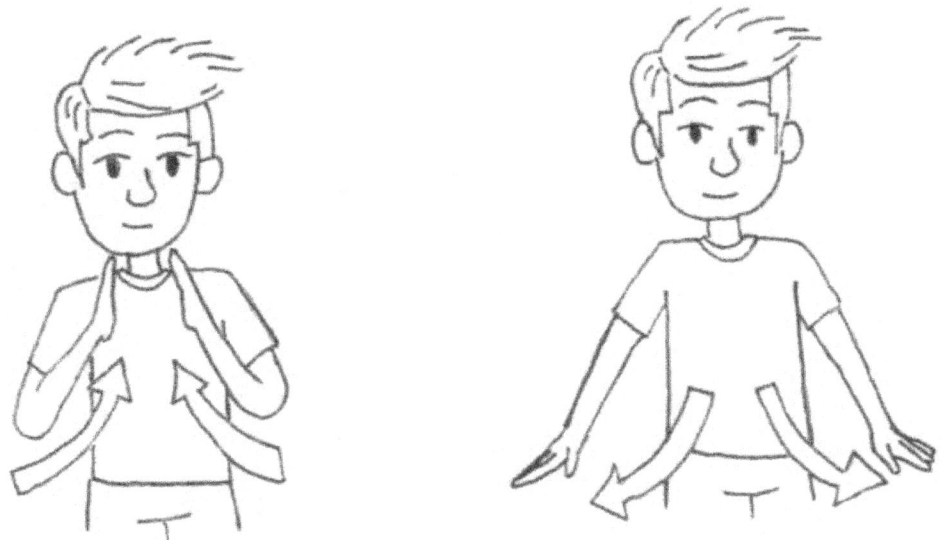

The next movement is called piano. Your right hand is above the left hand just below the chest. Both palms are facing down. Bring your elbows in close to the body so the hands separate no wider than the shoulders and then bring them back to the original position. This helps the heart, lungs and builds yin energy in the body.

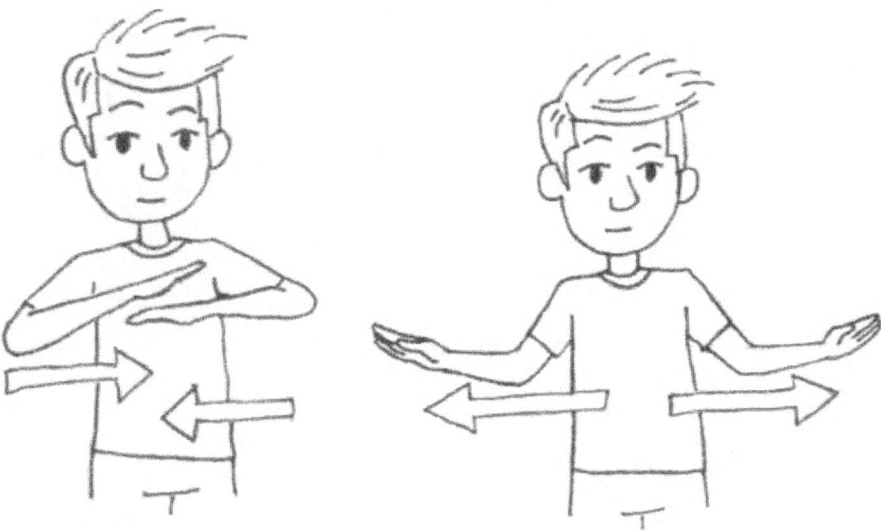

The next movement is called fish. It is the same as the previous one only the palms are turned up this time. This helps the heart, lungs and builds yang energy in the body.

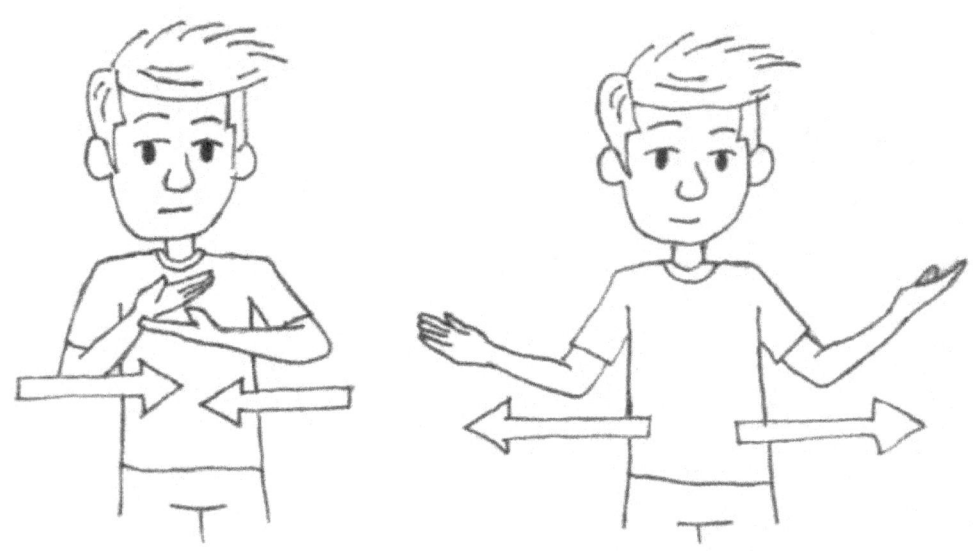

The next movement is called wind. The palms face each other a few inches apart and keeping the hands the same distance move them side to side; while keeping the elbows in close to the body. This helps the liver, spleen, kidney and balances both sides of the body.

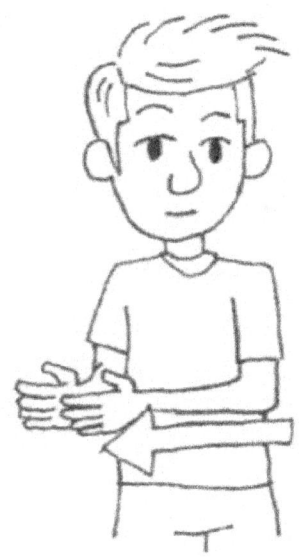 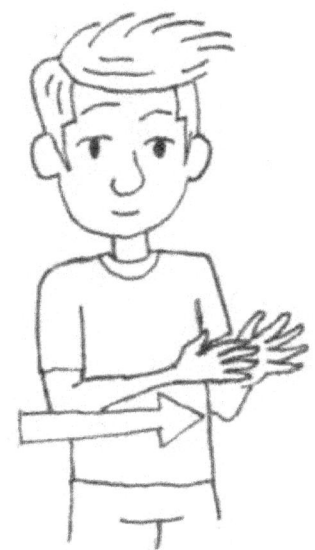

The next movement is called circle left and right. The palms stay a few inches apart and still keeping the elbows in close to the body circle the hands to the left and then to the right. This helps the liver, spleen and digestion.

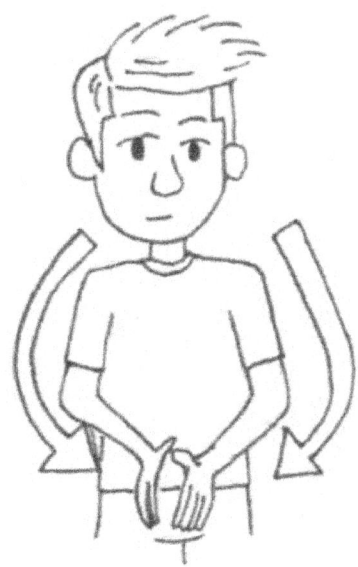

The next movement is called row. The hands form a "C" shape and imagine a ruler taped to the back of the hand and wrist so you can't bend the wrist. Keep the elbows in close to the body and move the hands like you were rowing a boat. This helps the stomach and to balance the yin and yang energies.

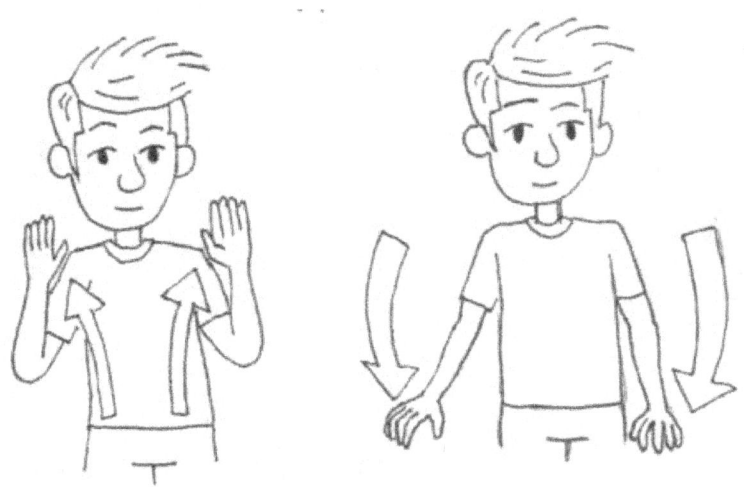

The next movement is called wheel. The right hand is at chest level and the left hand at the belly button. Circle the right hand forward and down as the left hand comes up to the chest level. Continue circling the hands forward down and up like a wheel rolling along.

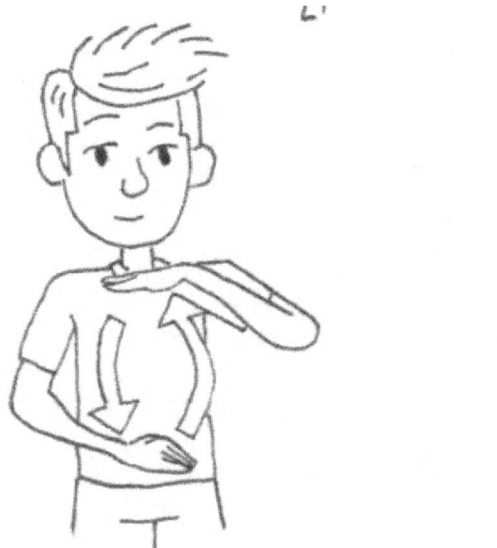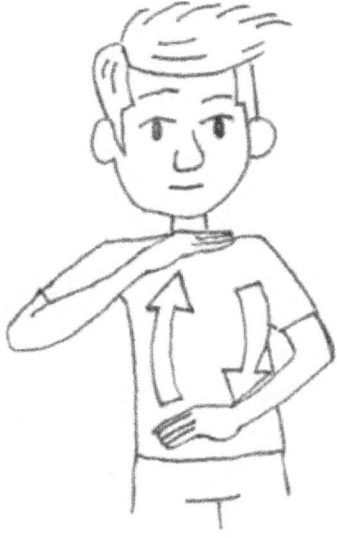

The next movement is called boat. Right hand above the left hand with the palms facing down. Keep right hand above the left as you move your arms side to side like a boat rocking in the water.

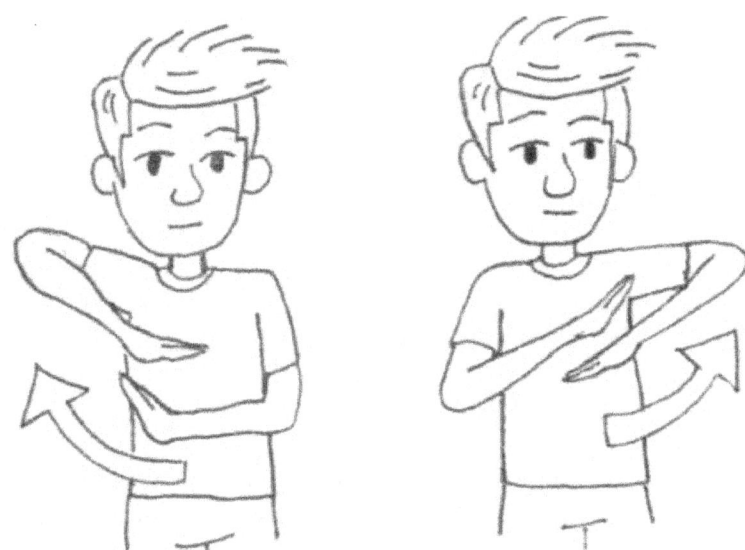

The next movement is called ear. The arms hang at the side palms facing in. Swing the arms up to the ears quickly and then slowly lower them back to the side. Make sure the center of the palm is close to the ear but not touching. About a half inch distance from the ear. This helps the kidney and with ear problems.

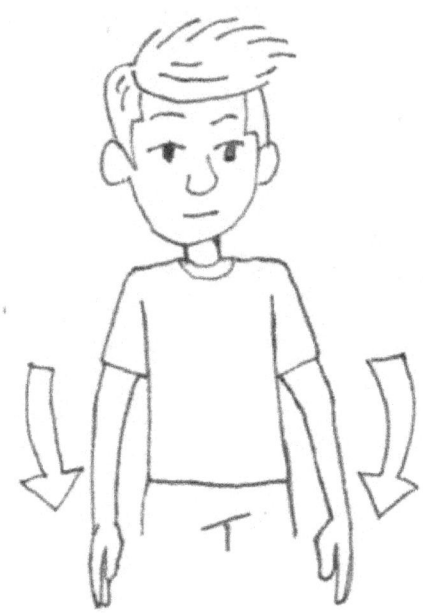
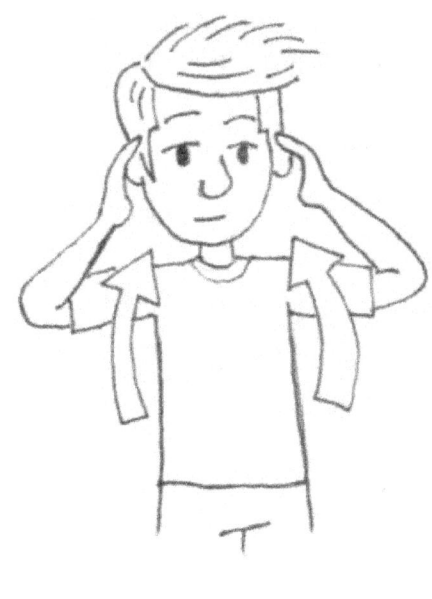

The next movement in the series is eye. The hands form a duck bill shape. The arms hang to the side like the previous movement. Swing the arms up in front of the eyes quickly so that you are looking through the duck bill. Not so close that you strike the eyes. Again slowly lower the arms to the starting position. This helps the liver and the eyes.

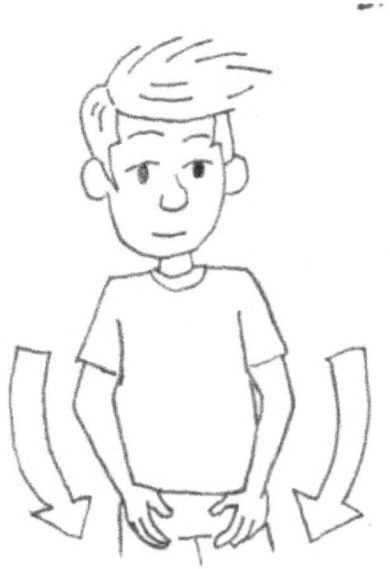
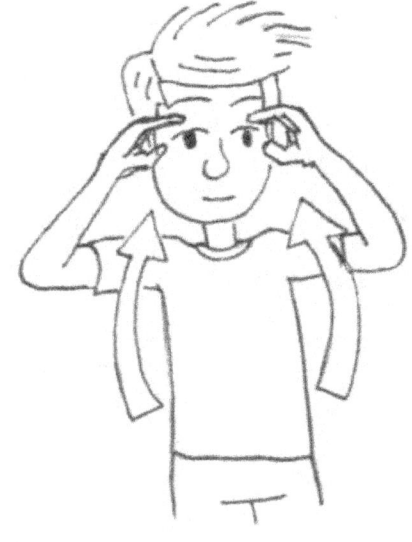

The next movement is called palm. The palms face the belly swing out to the sides and then back in again. This helps the kidneys and brings energy into the lower dantian.

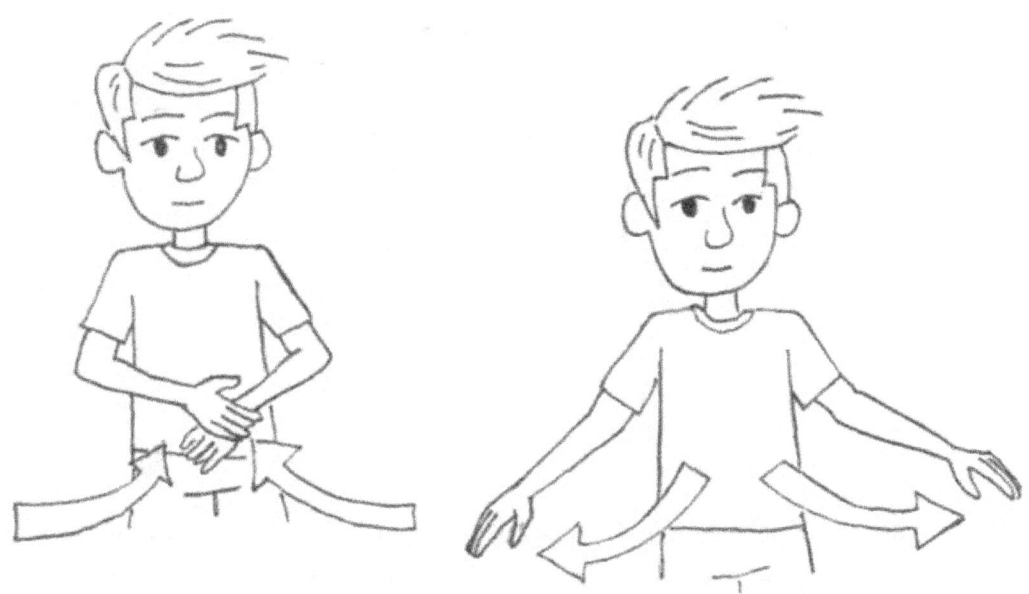

The close is the last movement in the series. Hold the hands together in front of the chest for about two to three minutes. Then let the hands drop to the side. Finish by lifting the arms up from the elbows with the palms facing down; while inhaling through the nose. Exhale through the mouth as you let the arms float back down. This balances the energy in the whole body and centers the mind.

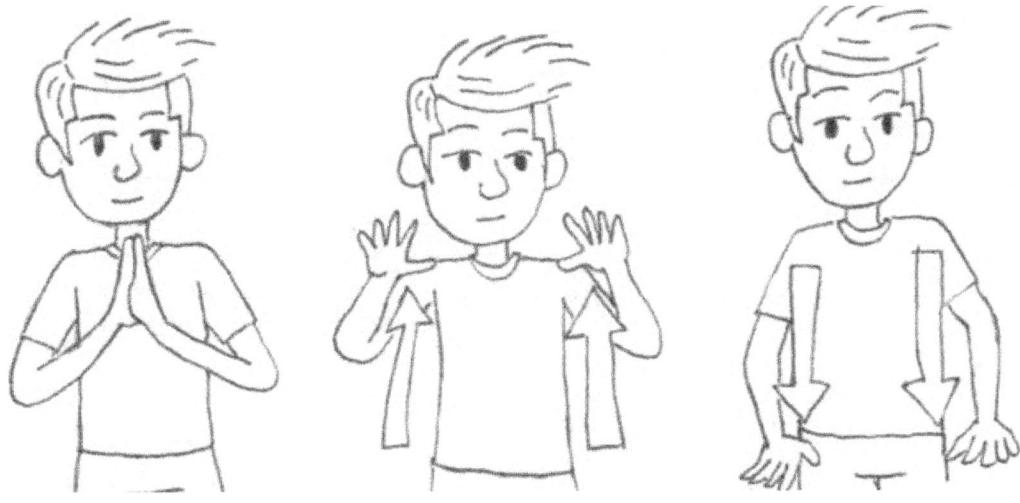

The exercises seemed easy to do but after doing them for a while I noticed that my arms and shoulders began to get heavy. What I liked the most about these exercises was that my grandparents learned them and I could practice the exercises with them.

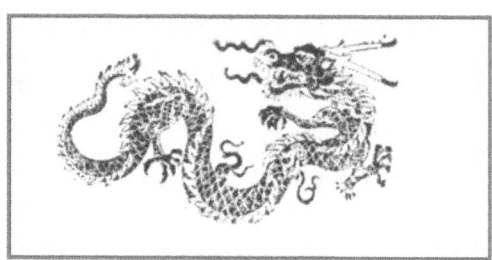

We then took a break and John invited me inside his house to have congee with him. I had no idea what it was but he explained that it was like a porridge only it was made with rice. It was easy to make and it was a good way to produce Qi and blood without stressing the digestive system. He reminded me that the Qi we get from food is called Gu Qi (Goo Chi).

This was the basic recipe that he used:

1 cup of rice

5-10 cups of water (depending on how thick you want it)

Cook 4-6 hours on a low flame.

When finished you can season it with salt, miso or honey.

John added fish and pork to his with some raw peanuts. I was not sure that I would like it but once I tasted it I knew it was something I would have to learn to make on my own. He then explained that congee can also be used for healing as well. The example he used was if someone had a cold. What he called a "Wind Cold". He said that you would add fresh ginger and scallions into the basic recipe and it would help to get rid of the chills, fever and scratchy throat. I remember thinking how much I had to learn.

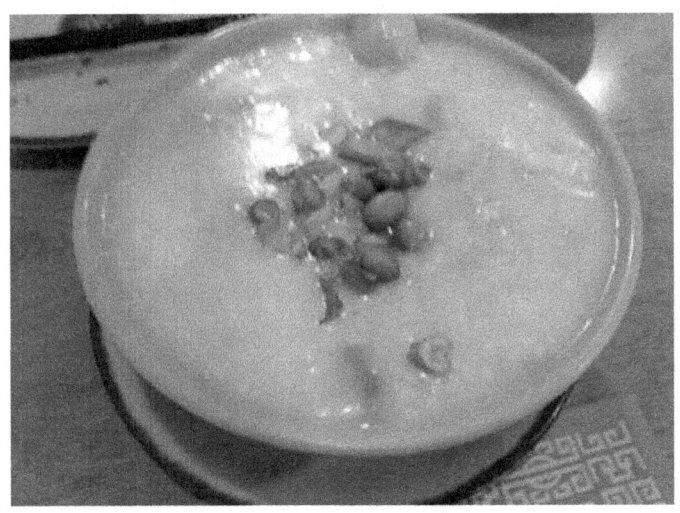

The day had gone by so fast and I had to go back to my grandparents and settle in for the evening. It was so much fun watching TV with them and doing the Fragrant Qigong exercises that we had learned.

As usual John wanted me to practice a whole week before he would teach me something new. He said it was a way of making sure I knew the exercises and that I was able to do them without him. I would have to do them on my own when I went back to Cleveland and he would not be there to guide me.

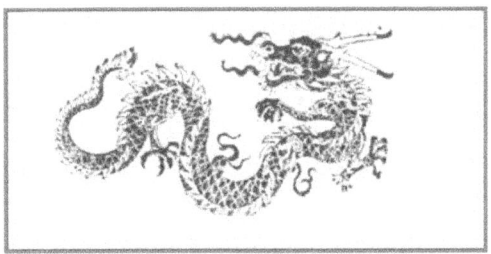

When a week had gone by I was back up the hill eager to see what John had in store for me. This day he was going to teach me a meditation called the "Inner Smile". This one was to be done sitting in a chair. I was to sit on the edge of the chair with the feet flat on the floor and the hands resting on the legs. I was to imagine that I was like a Christmas tree ornament with a string attached to the top of my head. This was to help lengthen the spine and open all the joints. The breathing was to be deep and slow.

I was then to imagine smiling into my forehead and eyes. John said to imagine it like a warm, healing light warming my forehead and eyes. Then I was to imagine the warm smiling energy flowing down my face, down the throat and into my heart. As I smiled into my heart I was to focus on the color red.

Then the smiling energy was to flow to the spleen on the left side of the boy under the ribs and behind the stomach. I was to focus on the color yellow.

From there I was to imagine the smiling energy going left and right into my lungs; while I focused on the color white.

From there the smiling energy was to flow to the back into the kidneys on each side of the spine and focus on the color blue.

Then the smiling energy was to go into the liver on the right side of the body just under the ribs. I was to focus on the color green.

I was to spend one to two minutes at each organ and then let the energy flow down into the lower dantian and store the energy there.

This exercise should take about fifteen minutes to complete and then allow the mind and body to slowly come back to my normal awakened state. I felt so relaxed after doing that meditation and it made me feel very happy at the same time. This would end up being one of my favorite meditations.

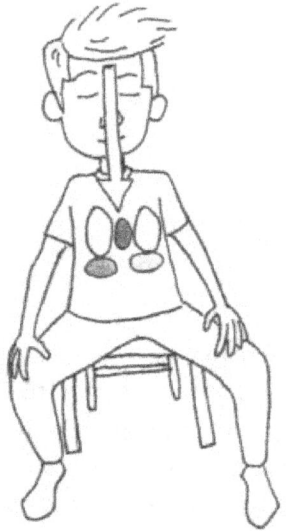
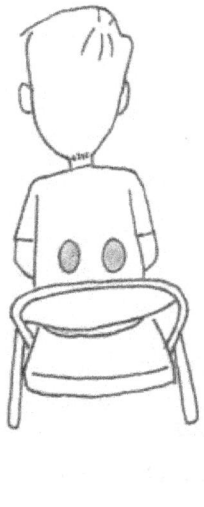

As usual, I was to practice for a week and then come back to learn more. It was not like I didn't see John at all during these times; he was always around doing things on my grandparent's house. So I would get to talk to him about everyday things. He always seemed at peace like nothing would ever bother him. It was calming just being around him.

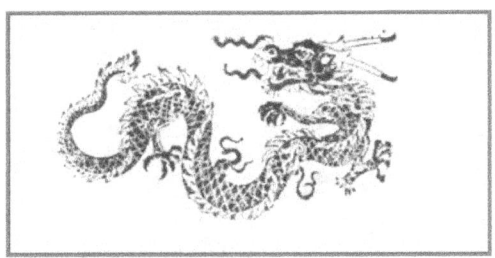

One day during the week he asked my grandparents if he could take me with him to Pittsburgh with him. He was getting a ride and was going to go to the China Town that was located there. He wanted to get some groceries from the Chinese supermarket and some herbs that he needed to make what he called a liniment.

The person we rode with dropped us off in the China Town area and said they would be back in a few hours to pick us up. It was located at the corner of Grant Street and the Boulevard of the Allies. John said it was small compared to New York's China town. There were a couple of restaurants, a Chinese supermarket and an herb store.

I was amazed at the supermarket. I had never seen anything like that before. So different than our grocery stores back in Cleveland. There was a section that had roasted ducks hanging, the whole duck, beak and all. Big hunks of roasted pork and something John told me was roasted pig intestines.

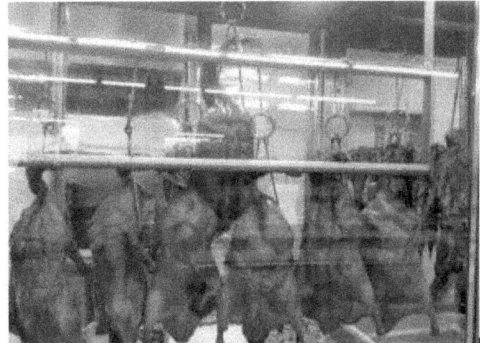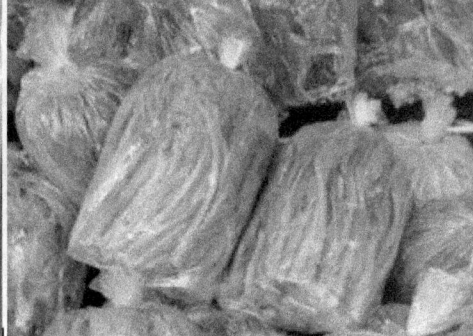

The vegetables were all laid out on counters with names like you choy, bok choy and ong choy. Fruits that had names like pomegranate, longan, lychee, and durian. The durian was big and had these spikes coming out of it. One was cut open and it stunk so bad and John said that was the smell of the fruit. John said it was good if you could get passed the smell.

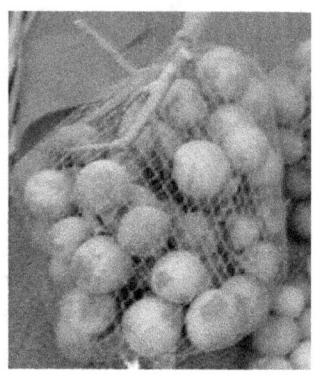

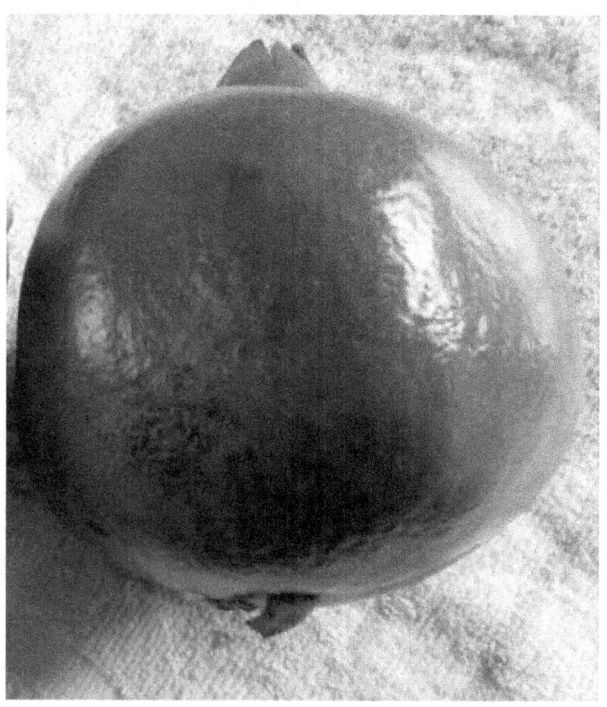

John had purchased a lot of vegetables and some rice. He bought very little meat and explained to me that meat was used for flavoring in Chinese cooking. The vegetables were the main dish with the rice. It was what he was used to eating and how he learned to cook from his mom.

We then went into the herb store where he picked up a lot of different herbs. These were the herbs he was going to use to make his liniment. They included angelica root, comfrey root, cinnamon bark, valerian root, hyssop, safflower petals and calendula. He told me these were American herbs as he could not find the ones he would have normally used if he was in China.

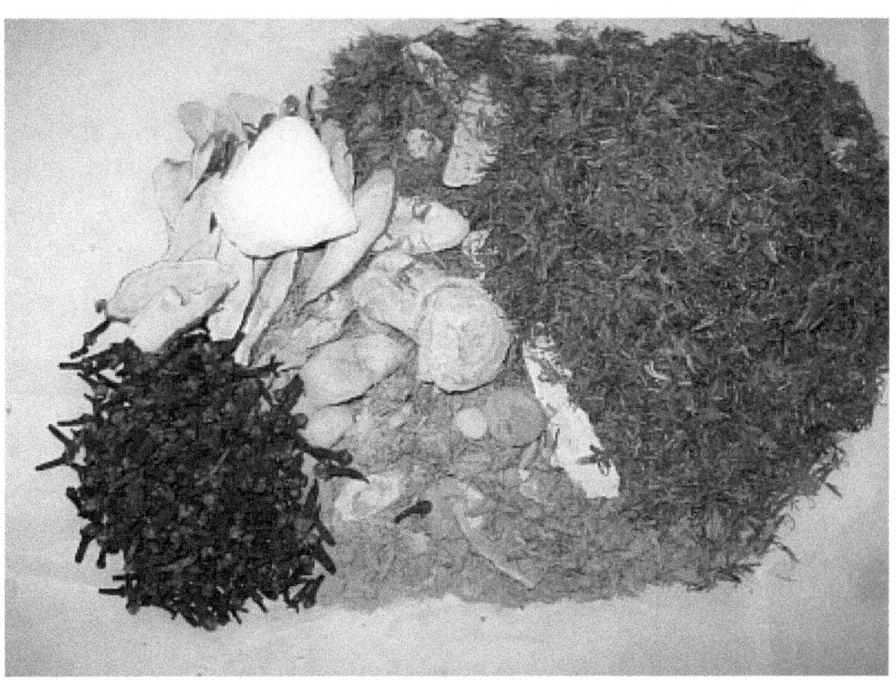

After leaving there we walked for about two blocks and came to a liquor store. I was shocked to see John go inside as I though he didn't drink any alcohol. When he came out he saw the look of disappointment on my face and then explained that the alcohol was to be used in making the liniment. The alcohol brings out the healing ingredients of the herbs and that is what is used for the liniment.

Our ride showed up and we got into the car and headed back to Smock. It was a good trip and I learned quite a bit.

During the ride home John began to explain to me about Yin and Yang. Yin and Yang need to be balanced. Balanced people respond better to stress. Yin is cool, internal, soft and flexible, and like stored energy. Yang is hot, external, hard and brittle, and is like moving energy. He explained to me that Yin and Yang were relative and it is one of theories used in Traditional Chinese Medicine.

He explained it by describing a candle. The candle itself if Yin, the stored energy. The flame is Yang the moving energy. You cannot have one without the other. If you had no candle you could not have the flame and if you had no flame you could not light the candle.

Yin people are quiet, pale looking, not physically strong and overwhelmed with too much activity. They tend to get more chronic illnesses and the illness creeps up and lingers for a long time.

Yang people are loud, physically strong and likes a lot of activities. They don't get sick very easily but when they do they get hit hard and recover very quickly. The illness comes on quick and goes away just as fast.

Even the organs in our bodies are either Yin or Yang. The Yin organs all store energy and they are the solid organs: heart, spleen, lungs, kidneys and the liver. The Yang organs are all hollow and the energy flows through them: small intestine, stomach, large intestine, bladder and the gall bladder. I had remembered that from last summer when I was with John.

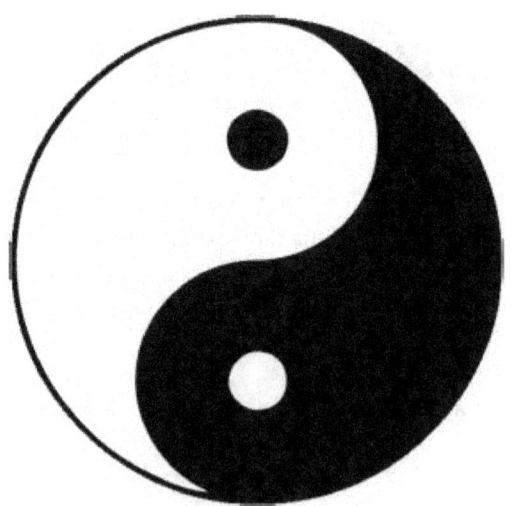

When we arrived back I helped John unload his groceries from the car. My grandparents had an old refrigerator that they kept in the garage for John to use. He put his meats and vegetables in there and took the rest up to his cabin. He placed his herbs in a cool dark cabinet he had until he was ready to use them. The rice he put in a cupboard and the fruits he left out on the counter top.

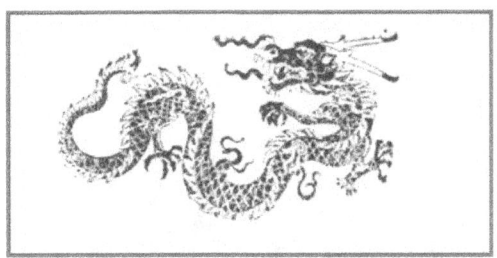

He then proceeded to teach me a new meditation called Yin and Yang Balance Meditation. I was to sit on a chair with my hands resting on my thighs and my knees at a ninety degree angle. My feet were to remain flat on the floor and the back straight and relaxed. The shoulders were to remain relaxed as well. I was to imagine roots growing out of the bottoms of my feet going into the ground and spreading out. And the sun shining brightly down on the top of my head.

I was to inhale and imagine drawing the yin energy of the earth up through my legs and going into the dantian. I was to simultaneously imagine the yang energy coming down from the sun and also going into the dantian. This was to balance both the yin and yang energies in my body. If one was out of balance I could just focus more on the one part of the meditation. John also mentioned that if I kept my palms turned up it would help build the yang and if I kept the palms turned down it would help build the yin.

As usual, the week went by with me practicing all that John had taught me up to that point. I was real excited to go up to see John that morning that I tripped over a tree root and my leg landed on a nice size rock just before reaching John's cabin. I was surprised how it started to bruise quickly.

John had noticed what had happened and came down to help me up. He had me walk to his cabin where he sat me down on a chair and brought out this big glass jar with all the herbs in it that he got from the Chinese market. It was filled with the herbs and the alcohol he bought too.

He took some of the liniment out of the jar and rubbed it on my bruise. It smelled almost as bad as the durian fruit at the market. John instructed me to leave it on for several hours and keep my leg up to rest it. He helped me back down to my grandparent's house for me to rest. After a couple of days my leg felt so much better and the bruise was almost gone. I as well as my grandparents were amazed.

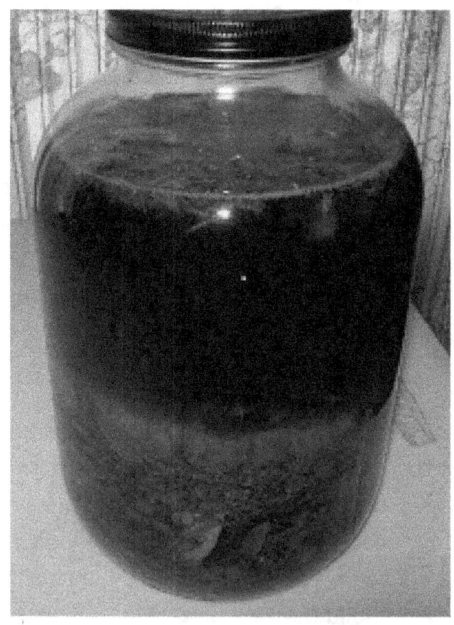

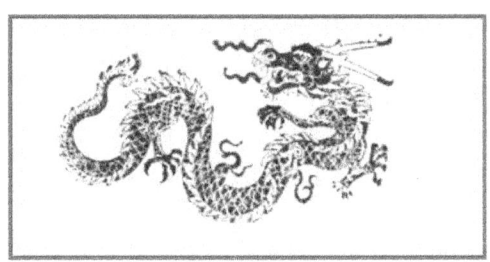

After resting for several days I went back up to see John to work with him and go over the exercises he had shown me up to that point. That day he told me he was going to show me some exercises to help with my eyes. He noticed I wore glasses and he mentioned the exercises would keep my eyes healthy. He called them Chinese eye exercises. There were seven exercises total. He made it clear that at no time was I to put pressure on the eyeball itself.

The first one I was to take my first and second fingers and put them together. Then I was to put the second finger at the edge of the nose on each side. Where my first finger ended up I was to push gently up and in for a count of eight.

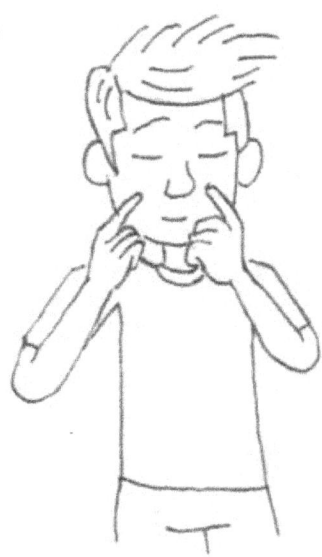

The second exercise was to bend both of my first fingers and then starting from the center right on the bone of the upper eye I was to go outward towards the end of the eye socket. Eight times and then repeat the same motion on the bottom.

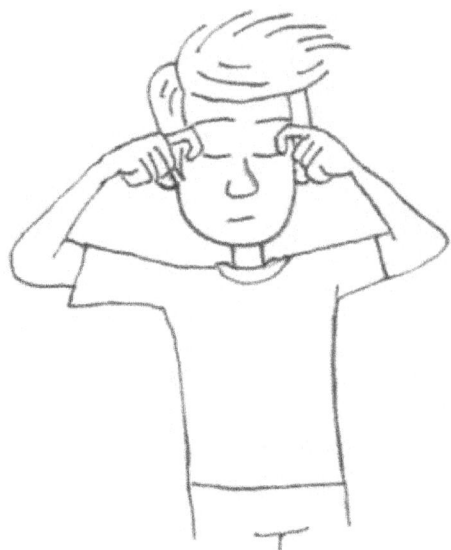

The third exercise was for me to put my thumb and index finger together and where the crease ended I was supposed to put the opposite thumb on top and the index finger on the bottom for support and massage with gentle pressure for a count of eight.

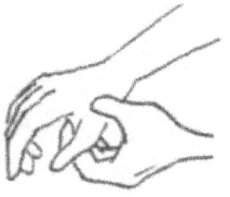

The fourth exercise I was to put my thumbs in the inner corner of the eyes and my finger tips at the hairline on the forehead. I was then to pretend my hands were like spiders doing push ups.

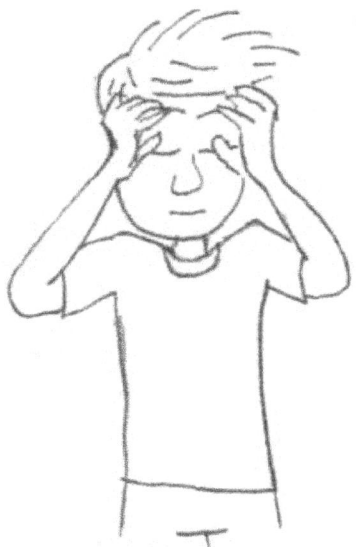

The fifth exercise was for me to take my first finger and start at the center and follow my eyebrows out to where they ended. In the soft spot there I was to press gently for a count of eight.

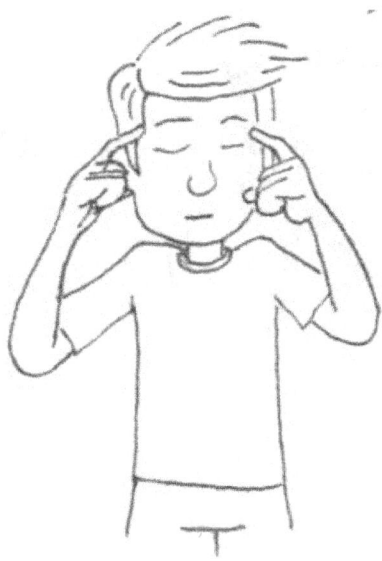

The sixth exercise was for me to take either hand and with my thumb and first finger pinch in the upper inner corners of the eye for a count of eight.

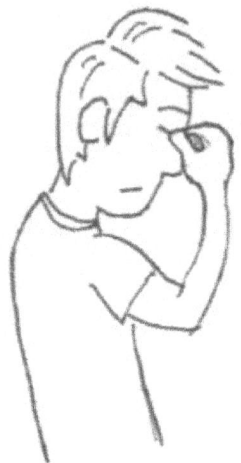

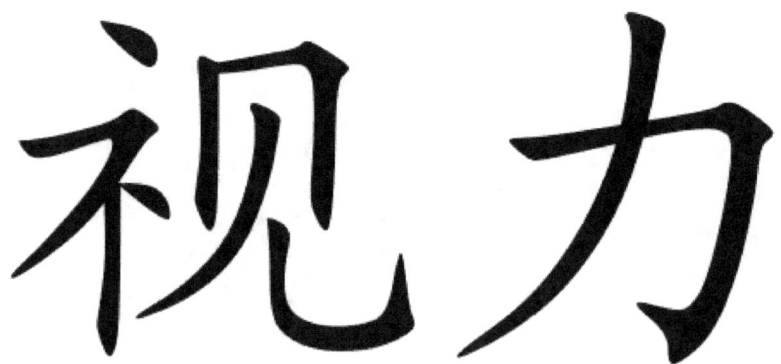

Vision

The seventh and last exercise was for me to imagine a giant clock in front of me. I was then supposed to look from 2 down to 8 ten times. Then I was to go from 10 down to 4 and following that by looking from 9 to 3. I was to finish by rolling my eyes 10 times going clockwise and then reversing the other way for 10 times. The finish was to rub the palms of my hands together briskly and then cover my eyes with my palms and let the warmth soak in the eyes.

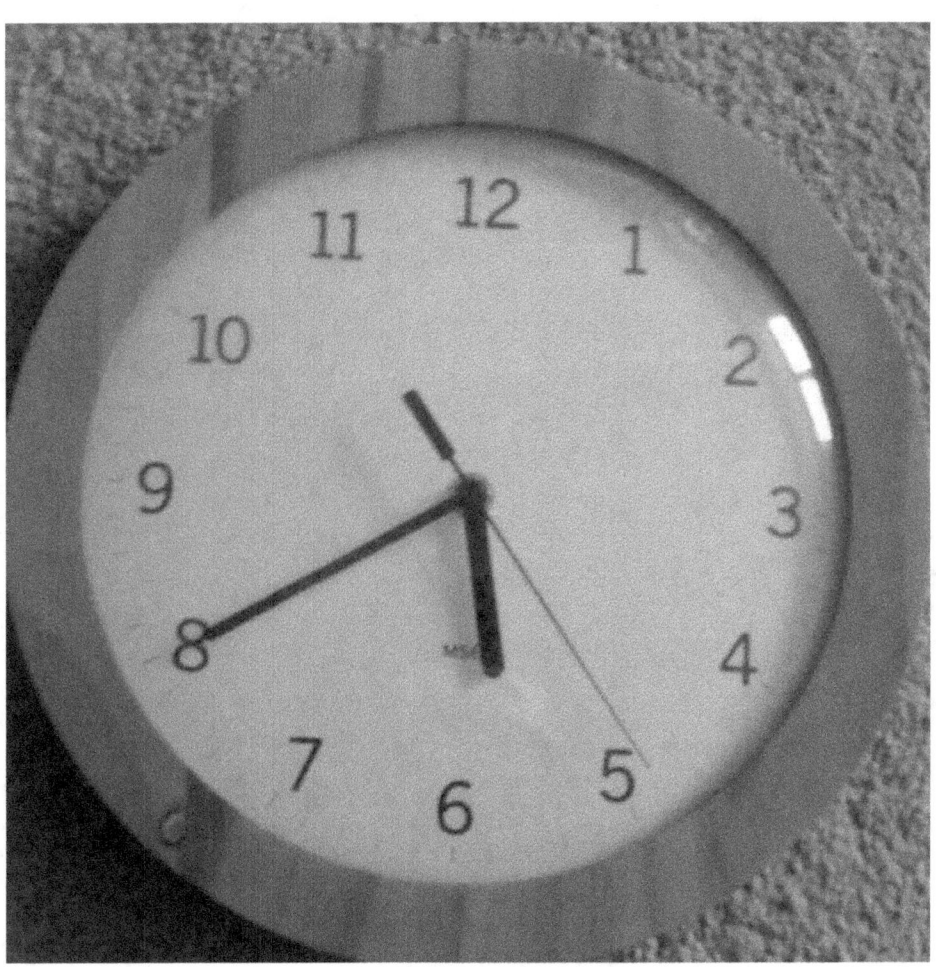

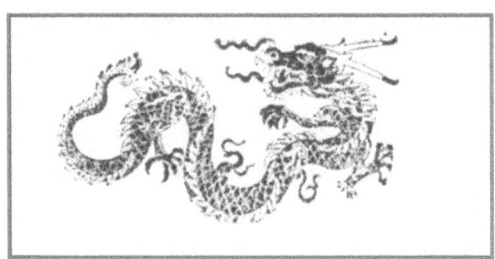

Another week of practicing and then I was going to learn more from John. I woke up as usual and had breakfast and was ready to go up the hill. When I walked out the back door there was John waiting for me. He mentioned that we were going to take a walk down to the reservoir and he was going to teach me about getting and working with the Qi of nature. It was about a mile and a half walk to the reservoir and John had wanted to get an early start.

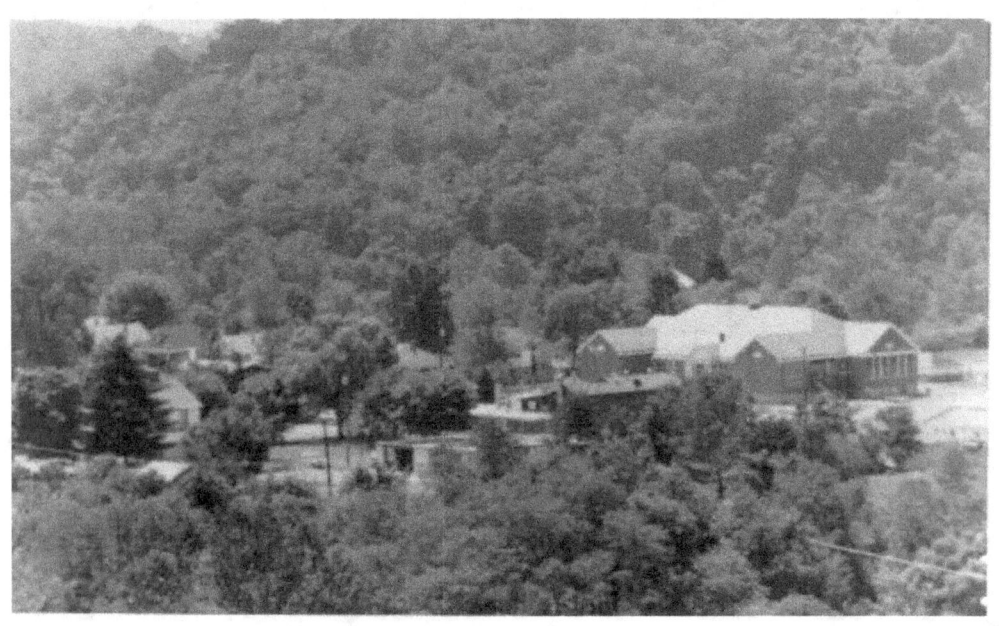

We started down the hill and John stopped at a natural spring that was flowing from a little mound that was right at the road up to the hill. He had an empty jug with him that he used to collect the water so we could take it with us.

As we walked along the road to the reservoir he began to tell me about gathering the Qi of the earth. Trees and plants take in the air we breathe, the minerals and water from the ground, and the light from the sun. When the Qi from the universe mixes with the energy from the earth it becomes a powerful energy source. He told me that in Chinese history the Chinese have used trees, bushes and flowers for healing medicine.

Trees absorb and transform negative, toxic Qi into clean healthy Qi. Working with trees is done to remove stale Qi from the meridians, tonify the internal organs and replenish Qi in the body. It also nourishes the blood and helps to strengthen the nervous system. Bushes are the same as trees but they do not have the powerful Qi that trees do.

Flowers stimulate the nervous system and the colors and shapes can affect the emotions of a person. The colors can be absorbed into the organs. He reminded me of last summer when we talked about the five elements and the colors that represent the internal organs.

Mountains, valleys and deserts gather the energy released from the sun. These energies are released a lot faster than the energy of oceans, lakes and streams.

Oceans, lakes and streams release the sun's energy slowly and it is important in cultivating the Qi. Our bodies can instantly absorb the energy from water. Herbal teas are a form of energized water that helps with a person's body.

When we finally reached the reservoir we sat for a moment just to enjoy the sun and our surroundings. He explained that the Qi was everywhere and we just needed to learn how to absorb it. John had started me on how to gather Qi energy from a tree. He explained that trees are like us; they stand upright like us and they drink water through their roots and require sunlight just like us.

He instructed me to find a healthy tree, any type to begin with. John said that the principle to absorbing the Qi is intent and breath, to draw the healing Qi from any natural source.

First face the tree and close the eyes and feel the presence of the tree. Then inhale through the nose and intend for the healing Qi of the tree to enter the body. Exhaling the stale, negative, toxic Qi from the body. This I was to do for several minutes.

Then I was to imagine the energy of the tree flowing from its leaves into the top of my head, what John had called the Bai Hui point, an acupuncture point on the crown of the head. Then I was to imagine the Qi flowing down through my body, out through my feet and being absorbed by the roots of the tree. I was to imagine flowing up the tree like sap and reaching all the way up to the highest branches. And then repeating for several times.

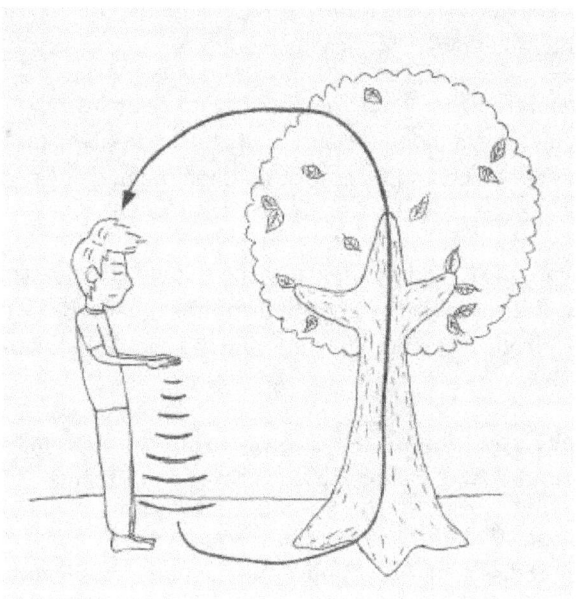

After doing that for several moments I was to reverse the flow and let the Qi flow from the roots of the tree up through my feet into my body and then out the crown of the head into the leaves of the tree. I was to do that several times. I was to imagine a constant stream of Qi flowing between me and the tree.

John told me that over time he would teach me how to do the same with flowers, bushes, mountains, lakes and streams. Each one is different and may need some different techniques. This was exciting to me in two ways; one, John was going to teach me how to gather energy from these areas of the earth. Second it meant he was going to continue teaching me year after year. I was very excited.

I practiced this exercise for a week and after a few days I started to imagine myself as a tree with roots sinking deep within the ground and my upper body like leaves reaching up to the sky.

It was almost August and I would be going home in about four weeks and I was wondering if John was ever going to teach me the Tai Chi 24 form. I didn't have to wait long as the next morning John said he was going to begin teaching me the form.

He went over the forms and their names as he began to teach me.

1. Beginning Form (Opening Movement) (drawings 1-3)
2. Part the Wild Horse's Man on both sides (drawings 4-7)
3. The White Crane Spreads its Wings (drawings 8-9)
4. Brush Knee and Twist Step on both sides (drawings 10-12)
5. Hand Strums the Lute (drawings 13-15)
6. Step Back and Whirl the Arms on both sides (drawings 15-18)
7. Grasp the Bird's Tail left side (drawings 19-21)
8. Grasp the Bird's Tail right side (drawings 22-24)
9. Single Whip (drawings 25-27)
10. Wave Hands Like Clouds (drawings 28-30)
11. Single Whip (drawings 31-34)
12. High Pat on Horse (drawing 35)
13. Kick with Right Heel (drawing 36)
14. Strike Opponent's Ears with Both Fists (drawing 37)
15. Turn and Kick with Left Heel (drawing 38)
16. Push Down and Stand on One Leg, left Side (drawing 39)
17. Push Down and Stand on One Leg, right Side (drawing 40)
18. Fair Lady works the Shuttle both sides (drawings 41-42)
19. Needle at the Bottom of the Sea (drawing 43)
20. Flash the arms (drawing 44)
21. Turn Deflect Downward, Parry and Punch (drawing 45)
22. Apparent Close Up (drawing 46)
23. Cross the Hands (drawing 47)
24. Closing Form (closing movement) (drawing 48)

1

2

3

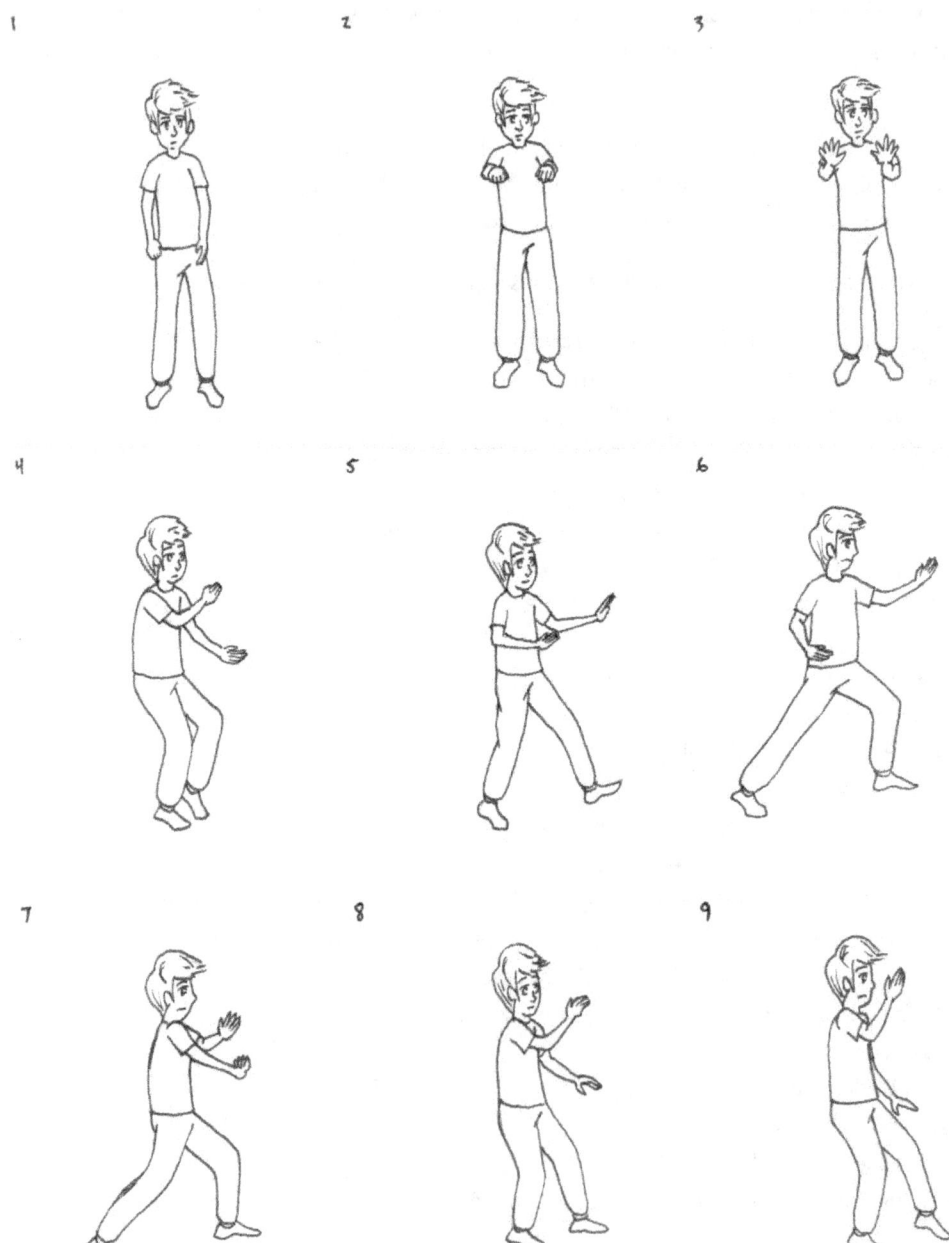

4

5

6

7

8

9

10

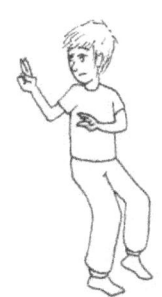

11

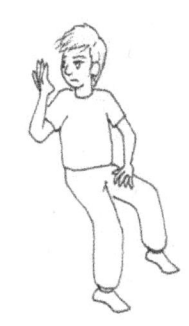

12

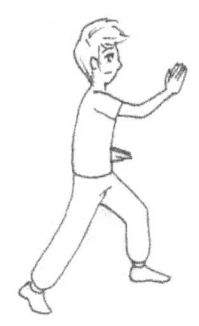

13

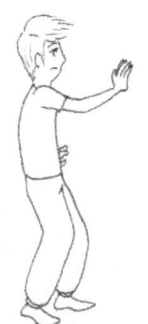

14

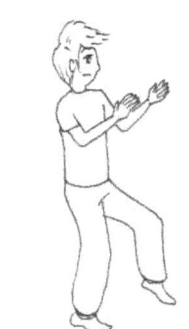

15

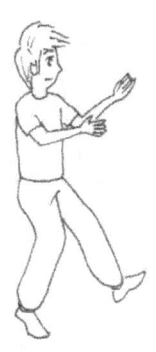

16

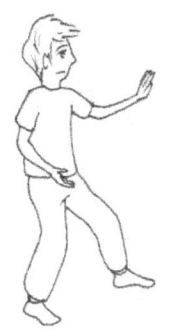

17

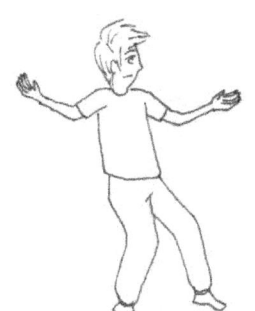

18

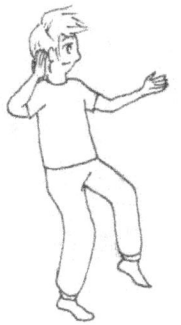

19

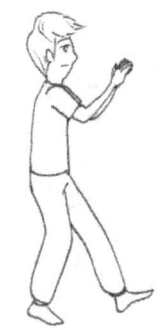

20

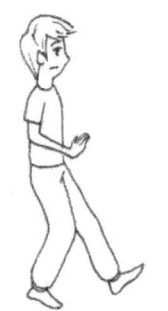

21

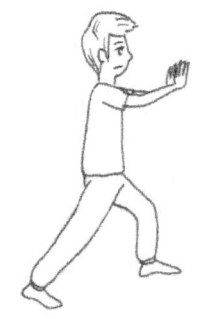

22

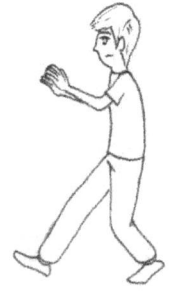

23

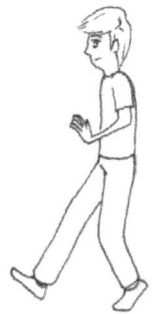

24

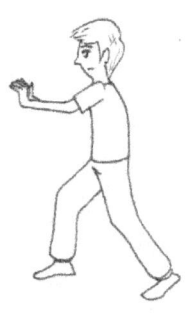

25

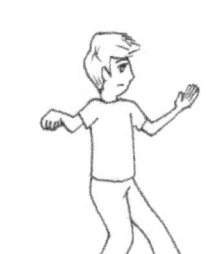

26

27

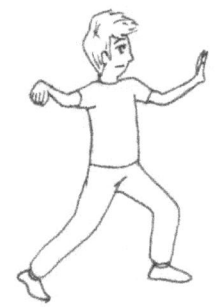

28

29

30

31

32

33

34

35

36

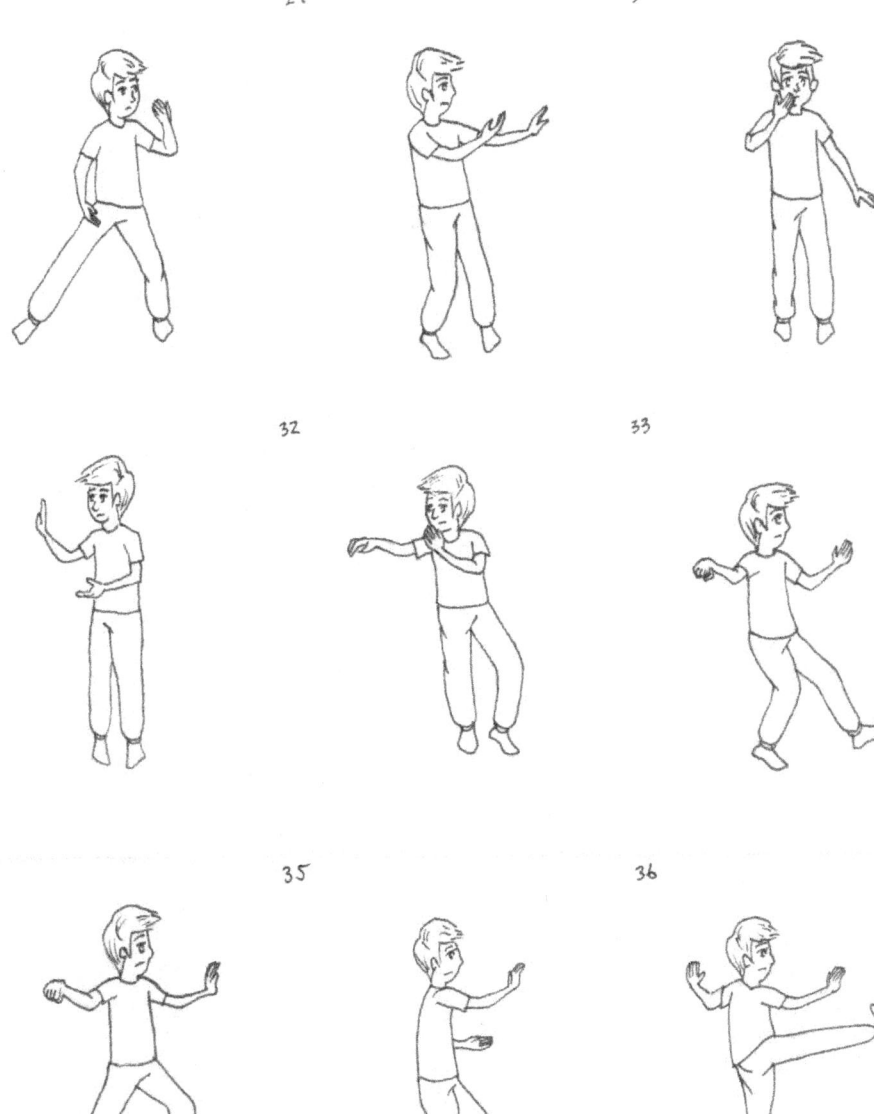

37

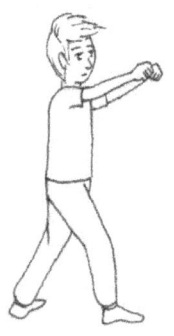

38

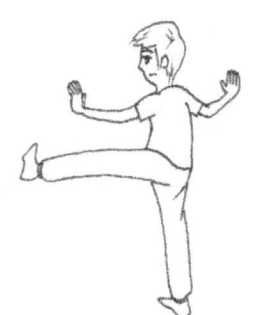

39

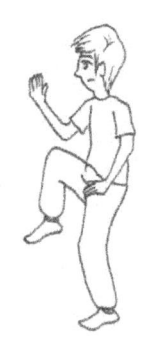

40

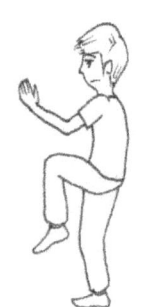

41

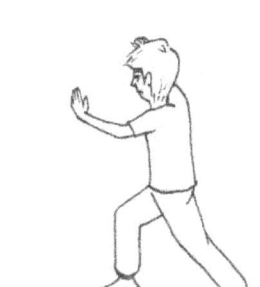

42

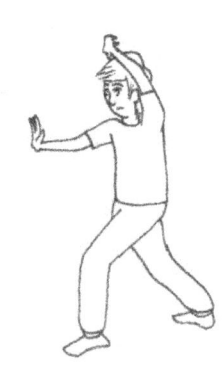

43

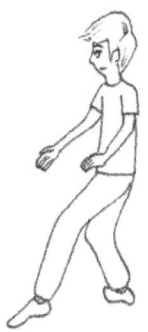

44

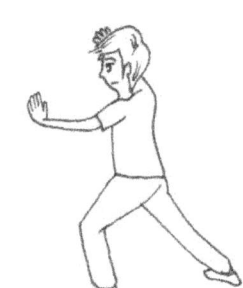

45

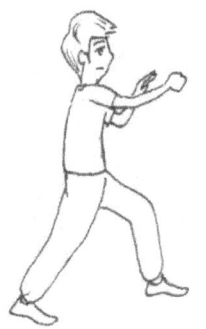

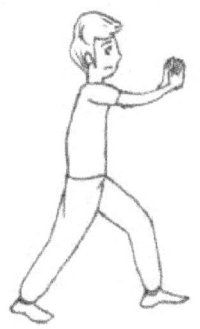 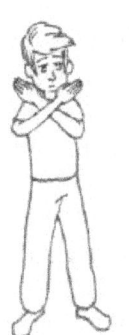 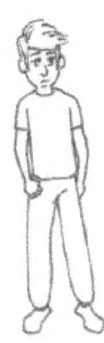

1) Beginning Form - Stand with your feet shoulder with apart and the body relaxed. Shift your weight to your right leg as you bend both knees bringing your left foot onto the ball of the foot. Step with your left foot wider than your shoulders and adjust the weight so that it is centered over both legs. Let your arms float up to the shoulder level with the palms facing down. Gently bend your legs as if you were sitting on a stool and resting your arms on a table. Slide your left foot to the right (left foot on the ball) as your left hands drops to just below your navel and your right hand above your navel and just below your breast bone (like you were holding a beach ball in front of your belly).

2) Parting the Horses Mane – Step with your left foot out to the side and back ninety degrees. Your left hand comes out and your right hand drops to your right hip with the palm facing down. Your left arm looks as if you were giving someone a one-armed hug. Shift your weight back and turn your left foot out forty five degrees and then shift your weight to your left leg bringing your right leg forward to the left and your right hand dropping to the bottom like you were holding a ball. Step with your right foot as your right arm comes out parting the horse's mane and your left hand drops to hip. Your right arm like you're giving a hug. Shift your weight back and turn your right foot out forty five degrees and slide your left foot forward towards your right and your left hand dropping to the bottom like you're holding a ball. Then repeat the beginning part by stepping with your left foot again and part the horse's mane.

3) The White Crane Spreads its wings – Slide your right foot to the heel of your left foot and then shift your weight to your right leg and bring your left foot up on the ball of your foot. Your left hand drops pointing to the floor at a forty-five degree angle and your right hand pointing up at a forty-five degree angle. Turn your waist to the left and then drop your right hand as your left hand comes up. Now turn your waist back to the right.

4) Brush Knee Twist Step – Now raise your left leg as your right hand rises up to your shoulder. Your left hand brushes your left knee as you step forward with your left foot and your right hand extends forward about seventy percent. Shift your weight back and turn your left foot out forty-five degrees and at the same time have your right palm turn to face you. Lift your right leg as your left hand rises up to your shoulder. Your right hand brushes your right knee as you step forward with your right leg and extend your left hand forward about seventy percent. Repeat on the left side again.

5) Strumming the Lute – Bring your right foot to the heel of your left foot. Shift your weight to your right leg as you extend your left foot forward onto the heel. Your left hand raises up the center of your body as your right hand meets your left and then drops downward and circles back and up. Both hands are now at head level and the palms facing inward towards your head. You turn your head to look behind you.

6) Turning and Whirling the hands on both sides – Turn and look forward and as you step back with your left foot your left hand faces up and you start to pull your left hand back as your right hand starts to come forward like you are pushing something out of your left hand. Look back and then turn and look forward. As you step back with your right foot, your right palm faces up and pull your right hand back as your left hand comes forward like you are pushing something from your left hand. Look back and then turn and look forward and repeat the same movements with your left leg and hand.

7) Grasping the Bird's tail left side – As you step back with your right foot your left hand comes forward like you are pushing something out of your right hand but the right hand stops just in front of the body and when your left hand reaches the fingertips of your right hand the hands drop and circle up to chest level. Your left arm is at ninety degrees palm facing in and your right hand is behind your left, palms facing, and the right fingertips are pointing up. Imagine holding a bird in the hand. Step diagonally towards the corner and extend the hands about seventy percent. Extend the hands forward with the palms facing down and then roll them back towards you about head level. Drop your hands to chest level and push the hands forward about seventy percent.

8) Grasping the Bird's tail right side – Turn your left foot forward as you turn your body and hands to face the opposite corner. Drop your hands and pull them towards you as you circle them up to the chest level. At the same time pull your right foot back to your left resting on the ball of the foot. Extend your hands with your right hand at a ninety degree angle and your left behind your right with the fingers pointing up. Imagine holding a bird in your hands. Step diagonally towards the corner and extend your hands out about seventy percent. Extend your hands out with the palms facing down and then roll them back towards the head. Drop your hands to chest level and push your hands forward about seventy percent.

9) Single Whip – Bring your left foot forward even with your right facing forward. Your hands at chest level circle around to the left side of the body. Drop your hands down and pull them in towards you at the same time sliding your left foot towards your right resting on the ball of the foot. Your left hand circles up to the eye, palm facing back. At

the same time your right finger tips come together at your right ear. Step straight to the left and extend your left hand out palm facing out. At the same time your right hand arcs back.

10) Waving the hands like clouds – Turn your left foot forward and come to the center, facing forward. Your right hand drops to the leg level with your palm facing in and your left hand face level with your palm facing in. As you slide your right foot to your left turn at the waist to the left and the arms follow the shoulders. Your left arm drops as your right arm comes up and step to the left as you turn the waist to the right. Repeat two more times and stop in the center.

11) Single Whip – Step with your left foot towards the corner and extend your left hand forward palm out and at the same time arc your right hand back with the fingertips together.

12) High Pat on Horse – Bring your right foot to the heel of your left foot and at the same time bring the back of your right hand into your left palm keeping the knees bent. Arms are to be at shoulder level.

13) Right Heel Kick – Reach up overhead with both hands and as you circle them down the outside bend both knees. When the hands cross over your right knee lift your leg and hands at the same time. Execute a right heel kick as the hands go out diagonally at forty five degree angles.

14) Double Ear Strike – Step with your right foot then shift your weight back as you reach back with both hands making fists. Bring your hands from the outside to the center executing a double ear strike.

15) Left Heel Kick – Pull your hands in toward your chest as you shift your weight back and rotate the waist to the left. At the same time rotating your right foot on the heel. As you turn to face the opposite corner slide your left foot over. As you reach up overhead sliding your right foot to the left and shifting the weight from your left foot to the right. Circle the hands down the outside and when they cross over your left knee raise the hands with your knee. Execute a left heel kick as the hands go out diagonally at forty five degree angles.

16) Push Down Standing on One Leg Left Side – Step with your left foot as your heels make a ninety degree angle keeping the weight centered over both legs. Shift to your right leg and bring your left hand to your right ear as your right hand slides to the hip. Drop down your right leg and shift the weight forward as your left hand goes forward lifting your right leg and hand as your left hand comes to the breast bone.

17) Push Down Standing on One Leg Right Side – Step with your right foot as your heels make a ninety-degree angle, keeping your weight centered over both legs. Shift to your left leg and bring your right hand to your left ear as your left hand slides to the hip. Drop down your left leg and shift your weight forward as your right hand goes forward lifting your left leg and hand as your right hand comes to the breast bone.

18) Fair Lady Works the Shuttles – Step forward with your left foot as your hands drop to the center like you are holding a ball with your right hand on the bottom. Bring your right foot to the heel of your left foot and step to the corner as your right arm rises to the forehead with the palm out and your left hand extending forward with the palm out. Shift the weight back to the center with your left hand on the bottom and bring your left foot to the right. Step with your left foot to the corner as your left arm rises to the forehead palm out and your right hand extends forward with the palm out.

19) Needle at The Bottom of The Sea – Bring your right foot to the heel of your left as you turn slightly to the right and shift the weight to your right leg as your left foot raises on the ball. At the same time your left hand drops to just above your left knee with the palm facing down and your right two fingers coming up to your right temple. As you bend your knees with the back straight your right hand comes down the side of the body.

20) Flash the Hands – Bring the hands to the chest as you slowly rise up and step with your left foot forward as you extend your hands forward with the palms facing out and your left arm at a ninety-degree angle and your right just below the left with the fingers pointing up.

21) Downward Parry, Block and Strike – Turn your left foot towards your right as you turn your waist to the right and your right foot rotating forty five degrees to the right. Your right arm extends straight out as your left hand comes to your right shoulder to block. Your right hand executes a downward parry towards the center of your body and then making a fist with your right hand. Bring your right hand to your right hip as you finish turning forward raising your left leg up. Step with your left foot and execute a right punch over top of your left hand. Your right palm facing up and your left palm facing down.

22) The Apparent Close Up – Extend both hands out with the palms facing up and as you shift your weight back, drop the hands downward and back. When your hands reach the body bring them up to the chest and then push forward shifting the weight forward.

23) Crossing the Arms – Turn your left foot towards your right and as you reach up over head with both hands rotate your right foot on the heel. As you circle the arms down

the outside sliding your right foot toward your left keeping the feet shoulder width apart. Cross the arms in the center and then reach up overhead with both hands.

24) The Closing Form – As you circle the hands down the outside bringing your feet together and your hands resting at your side.

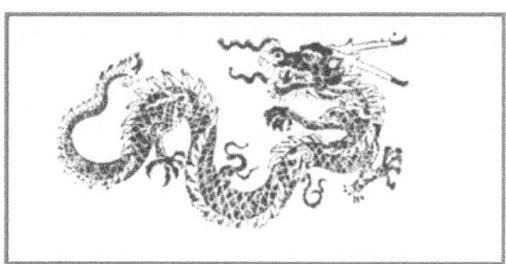

The entire month of August was spent learning the Tai Chi 24 form and reviewing the Qigong exercises and meditation that John had taught me. Even the ones from last year. The month seemed to have gone by so fast and before I knew my mom and dad had arrived to take me home. We would spend the weekend with my grandparents and leave on Sunday afternoon.

And just like last summer I was sad to leave my grandparents and John. I had learned so much from him over the last two summers and I knew there was so much more to learn. On Sunday afternoon we had said our goodbyes and got into the car and headed back to Cleveland.

After a few days of shopping for school supplies it was time to head back to St. Stanislaus where I was entering the sixth grade. My confidence was so much better than previous years and I was now talking more to my classmates and the teachers as well. I even began to talk more to the girl that I had the crush on.

It was the beginning of November and Thanksgiving would be here soon and then after that Christmas. It was always a fun time with my family at the holidays. There were so many traditions that we had grown up with and it may the holiday's all the more special.

On Sunday November sixth we were awakened by a phone call from my aunt in Smock; my grandfather had passed away the night before from a heart attack and my mom and dad were saddened by the news. It appeared that we would be going back to Smock, sooner than I had thought, only this time it was a sad occasion.

On the day of the funeral I remember holding my dad's hand while we were at the cemetery and when I looked up I could see my dad crying. It was the first time I had ever seen my dad cry and I felt very sad.

Two days later we were back on the road to Cleveland and everyone in the car was very quiet. As we drove passed the cemetery I could see where my grandfather was buried. It was then that I saw John standing at the grave with a sad look on his face. My grandfather was very kind to him and he was just as kind to my grandparents. It was then that it hit me; what would happen to John? Would he be able to stay? Would my grandmother sell the house? Would I be able to come back and learn more from him? Questions I would have to wait until the following year to get answers to.

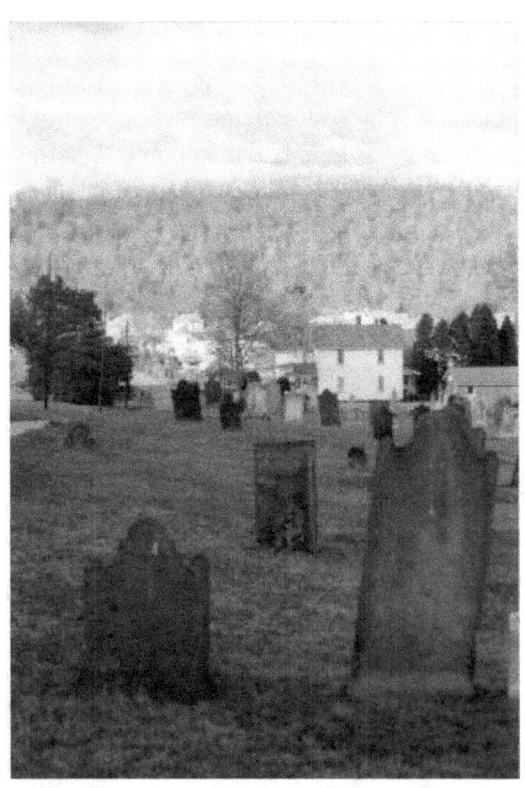

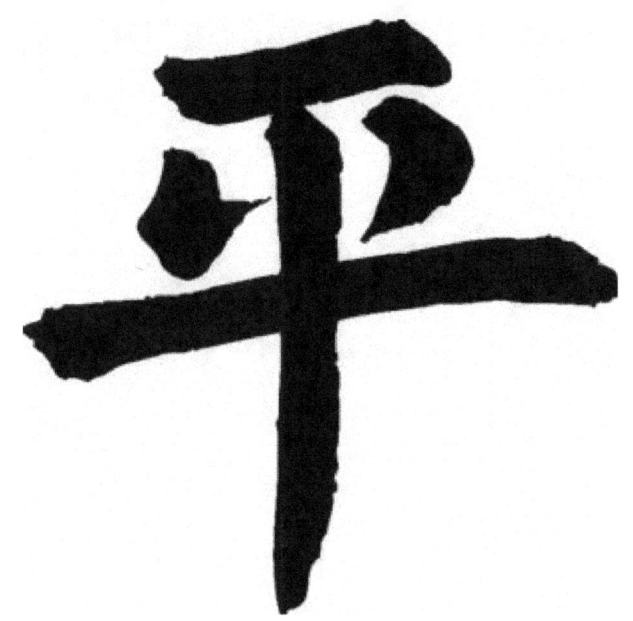

Peace